The Art of Making Perfume

How to Blend Essential Oils for Lasting Fragrances

Rebecca Park Totilo

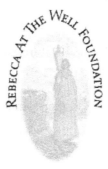

The Art of Making Perfume

Disclaimer Notice: The information contained in this book is intended for educational purposes only and is not meant to substitute for medical care or prescribe treatment for any specific health condition. Please see a qualified health care provider for medical treatment. We assume no responsibility or liability for any person or group for any loss, damage or injury resulting from the use or misuse of any information in this book. No express or implied guarantee is given regarding the effects of using any of the products described herein.

ISBN **978-0-9827264-1-9**

Table of Contents

Acknowledgements to the Lord

Song of Solomon 1:3-4 says, "Because of the savour (fragrance) of thy good ointments thy name is as ointment poured forth, therefore do the virgins love thee. Draw me, we will run after thee."

It is the sweetness and power of the Lord's fragrance that draws us to him. Like bees attracted to a flower, He captivates us by sending forth His sweet fragrance of love and forgiveness, causing His bride (of Christ) to desire and look upon him - being conscious of only Him.

His name, like an ointment poured forth, represents the whole nature and character of the one to whom it belongs - Yahweh in the flesh. And, with Yeshua's life poured out, contained no longer in Heaven, His mercy, grace, righteousness and power have reached out unto mankind.

Those who are found intoxicated by His fragrance have a deep desire awakened within them to run after Him, annulling all other worldly matters.

Introduction

Department stores filled with a myriad of fragrant aromas know how much women love perfume. Researchers believe women find perfume irresistible because of the scent's or perfume's ability to trigger an increase in the production of pheromones in their bodies.

In addition to a perfume's capability to help enhance a woman body's pheromones levels, they are appealing to women because of the attention they get from a member of the opposite sex or even from another woman. Many women will tell you that the reason they purchase a particular perfume is that it makes them feel better about themselves. It also makes them feel a bit more feminine. Not only does smelling great make a woman feel good about herself, but it will also make her feel attractive.

In studies carried out, nearly 80% of all women will make a perfume purchase at least once each year. Its no wonder since perfumes are made to attract the customer via the olfactory system (sense of smell) in order to persuade people to buy the perfumes or perfume-laced products (women's magazines) they are producing.

In this book, we will be looking at ways to make your own perfume so that you can produce a scent which is uniquely you, distinct from any of those that you can buy in a store or over the internet.

History of Perfumery

Historical records reveal that people's use of scents, aromas, fragrances and essential oils have been used in almost every culture for millenniums. The Egyptians used aromatics in embalming, while the Greeks attributed sweet aromas to their gods by burning incense and the Babylonians perfumed the mortar with which they built their temples. In fact, Cleopatra, the Queen of Egypt drenched the sails of her ships with the most exotic fragrant essential oils so that their essences would herald her arrival along the banks of the Nile. The Hebrews scattered fresh leaves, twigs, and stems of fresh mint, marjoram and other herbs on the dirt floors of homes and synagogues. By walking on these, the fragrant essential oils would be released into the air. This practice was also common in the temple, where they sacrificed animals where the scent acted as a disinfectant as well as an air freshener.

Both the Assyrian's and Egyptians used scented oils. Because of this, the demand for the raw materials necessary to produce both fragrances and remedies led to the discovery of new ways to extract scents from the plants used. Such techniques as pressing, decoction, pulverization and maceration were developed and mastered by both the Assyrian's and the Egyptians. They even made attempts to produce essential oils by distillation. These methods will be discussed in the next chapter.

Slowly, the use of perfumes spread to Greece, where not only were they used in religious ceremonies, but also for personal purposes as well. When the Romans saw what the Greeks were doing, they began to use fragrances even more lavishly. There are many manuscripts that ascribed to how herbs were brought from all over the world to produce the fragrances they used.

After the Roman Empire fell, so the use of aromas for personal use declined. However, during the Middle Ages, perfumes again were used, this time only in churches in Europe for religious ceremonies and to cover the stench of disease and death which abounded at that time.

When trade with the Orient was reestablished at the beginning of the 13th Century, exotic flowers, herbs and spices became more readily available around Europe. Venice quickly became the center of the perfume trade. It was not long before perfumery soon spread to other European countries. The perfume trade then developed even further, as those returning from the crusades reintroduced perfume for personal use.

By the late 18th Century, the synthetic material for fragrances was being produced, which led to the beginning of perfumery in the modern age. Thus, with the introduction of synthetics, perfumes would no longer be exclusively used by the rich and famous. Now with synthetics readily available to produce perfumes, they could be made on a much larger scale, although natural oils were still being used to help soften the synthetics. Today, natural products still remain a very important part of the production of perfumes in modern formulations.

More and more people today are turning away from the industrial techniques of producing perfume, preferring to make it themselves. Most find it is not only easy to do, but a great source of pleasure and fun.

Ancient Art of Extracting Oils

According to Miriam Stead author of "Egyptian Life" the process of distillation using steam was not known for the extraction of essences but there were three techniques available for producing perfumes from flowers, fruits and seeds. She writes "There was effleurage the Saturation of layers of fat with perfume by steeping flowers in the fat and replacing them when their perfume was spent. In this way, the Egyptians were able to create creams and pomades.

The Original Coneheads

A popular form of pomade was the so-called cosmetic cone which was worn on top of the head. Those frequently represented in banqueting scenes worn not only by the guests but also by the servants. The cone was usually white with streaks of orange brown running from its top. The coloring represented the perfume with which the cone was impregnated. As the evening progressed the cone would melt and the scented oil run down over the wig and garment creating a pleasing scent and no doubt a sticky mess. Throughout the course of an evening it became necessary to renew the scent on the cones and the tomb scenes show servants circulating among the guests replenishing the perfumed cream.

A popular late-night comedy television show called "Saturday Night Live" use to include an skit of a family with Coneheads. I am sure the writers of this routine thought they were being original although 'cone shape' heads was all the rage in ancient Egypt.

The second process for creating perfume was maceration that is dipping flowers, herbs or fruits into fats or oils heated to a temperature of about 65 degrees Celsius. This technique is depicted in a number of tomb scenes. The flowers or fruits were pounded in mortars and then stirred into the oil which was kept hot on a fire. The mixture was sieved and allowed to cool. It might then be shaped into balls or cones or if liquid poured into vessels. An alternative process may have been to macerate the flowers in water, cover the vessel with a cloth impregnated with fat and boil the contents of the vessel until all the perfumes had evaporated, fixing them in the fat which was then scraped off the cloth. This technique is still used by Peoples living near the source of the Nile.

Thirdly, there was the possibility of expressing the flowers or seeds. This process was borrowed from the manufacture of wine and oil. The material to be pressed was placed in a bag with a stick attached to each end. The sticks were twisted by a group of workmen. This technique was not used often as most recipes specify either maceration or enfleurage."

How Essential Oils Are Produced Today

Producing essential oils continues to take a lot of work. It takes sixty thousand Rose blossoms to produce one ounce of Rose oil, whereas Lavender is easier to obtain and yields approximately 7 pounds of oil from two-hundred and twenty pounds of dried flowers. The Sandalwood tree must be thirty years old and over thirty feet tall before it can be cut down for distillation. Myrrh, Frankincense, and Benzoin oils are extracted from the gum resins of their respective trees. While citrus fruits such as Orange, Lemon and Lime are squeezed from the peel of their fruits. Cinnamon essential oil comes from the bark of the tree (and leaf) and Pine oil comes from the needles and twigs. Other flowers must be picked by hand early in the morning before the sun rises and heats up, evaporating the essential oil within its petals.

Hence, you can understand the variation in pricing of various essential oils on the market.

There is a variety of ways in which essential oils are extracted. The most common methods steam distillation, solvent extraction, expression, effleurage and maceration.

Steam distillation involves using steam to pull essential oils from the plant by suspending the plant material over water in a sealed container, which is then brought to the boil. The steam containing the volatile essential oil is run through a cooler, and when it condenses the liquid is collected. The essential oil appears as a thin film on top of the liquid, as water and essential oils do not mix. The essential oil is then separated from the water by collecting in a small vial and the water into a large vat.

Solvent extraction involves using little heat, in order to preserve the oil which would otherwise be destroyed or altered during steam distillation. Plant material is dissolved in a liquid solvent of hepane, hexane, or methylene chloride as a suitable perfume solvent, which absorbs the smell, color and wax of the plant. After removing the plant material, the solvent is boiled off under a vacuum to help separate the essential oil. This can be achieved since the solvent evaporates quicker, which leaves a substance called 'concrete.' The concrete is mixed with alcohol to aid in filtering the waxes. The next process is to distil the alcohol away, which leaves an 'absolute.' The word 'absolute' will appear on the label of some bottled essential oils although they still contain 2-3 per cent of the solvent, therefore are not considered pure essential oil.

Citrus oils is expressed rather than distilled. Within citrus fruits such as Orange, Lemon, Lime and Grapefruit the essential oil is located in little sacs just under the surface of the rind. The oils need to be squeezed out or expressed from the peels and seeds. This is achieved by letting the fruit roll over a conveyer that has small needles coming outpiercing the little oil pockets in the citrus rind. The oil runs out and is caught and filtered.

As mentioned before effleurage is an ancient method of extracting oils that is rarely used today because of its long, complicated and expensive process. Fragrant blooms were placed upon sheets of warm animal fat (or long sheets of vegetable fat) which absorbed the essential oil. As flowers are exhausted, they are replaced with fresh blossoms. This process is repeated until the sheet of fat is saturated with fragrance and is separated with solvents leaving only the essential oil.

Macerated oils are not pure essential oils as they are 'carrier' oils. Plant material is gathered and chopped, then added to either sunflower or olive oil. The mixture is stirred for a while, then placed in the sunlight for several days. This process transfers all of the soluble components in the plant material including the essential oil then is carefully filtered. This process leaves a carrier oil infused with essential oil.

Ancient Uses for Perfumes

In ancient times, essential oils and other aromatics were used for religious rituals, as well as for the treatment of illness and other physical and spiritual needs. According to the Essential Oils Desk Reference compiled by Essence Science Publishing, "Records dating back to 4500 B.C. describes the use of balsamic substances with aromatic properties for religious rituals and medical applications. The translation of ancient papyrus found in the Temple of Edfu, located on the west bank of the Nile reveals medicinal formulas and perfume recipes used by the alchemist and high priest in blending aromatic substances for rituals performed in the temples and pyramids. As well, Hieroglyphics on the walls of Egyptian temples depict the blending of oils and describe hundreds of oil recipes. Within these writings tell of scented barks, resins of spices, and aromatic vinegars, wines and beers that were used in rituals, temples, for embalming and medicine. Thus, the Egyptians were credited as the first to discover the potential of fragrance and were considered masters in using essential oils and other aromatics in the embalming process. They created various aromatic blends for personal use, placing them in alabaster jars – a vessel specially carved and shaped for holding fragrant oils. In fact, when King Tut's tomb was opened in 1922, 350 liters of oils were discovered in alabaster jars. Amazingly, because of the solidification of plant waxes sealing the opening of the jars, the liquefied oil was in perfect condition.

In the upper region of Egypt, a sect of Jews, called Essenes, were known for their healing arts and use of essential oils. Both Philo and Josephus writings indicated that at the period in which John the Baptist and Jesus were born, the Essenes were scattered over Palestine, numbering about four thousand souls. The Essenes or Therapeuts (used interchangeably) refer primarily to the art of healing which these devotees professed, as it was believed in those days that sanctity was closely allied to the exercise of this power, and that no cure of any sort could be imputed simply to natural causes. (Source: http://sacred-texts.com, http://bopsecrets.org)

The Holy Scriptures record over 1,035 references to aromatics, ointments, savors, fragrances, plants and incense-most implying essential oils. Twelve of the most highly-praised fragrances in the world mentioned in the Bible include: Frankincense, Myrrh, Spikenard, Hyssop, Cypress, Myrtle, Aloes, Sandalwood, Galbanum, Cinnamon, Cassia, and Onycha. Many were in the prescribed preparation of the Holy Anointing Oil and Holy Incense for Temple services, as well as for anointing and healing the sick. The people of the ancient world understood the importance of maintaining wellness and physical health, as well as the oils' ability to enhance their spiritual state of worship, prayer, and for the purification from sin. King David alluded to this in Psalm 51:7 when he wrote, "Purge me with hyssop and I shall be clean: wash me, and I shall be whiter than snow." While David's Psalm may have been speaking of a "spiritual purification" from his own sin of adultery with Bathsheba, today we know that the chemical constituents of essential oils including hyssop are able to penetrate the cell wall and transport needed oxygen and nutrients to the cell nucleus. Most essential oils can be absorbed through the skin or inhaled into the lungs where they then make their way into the bloodstream. The sense of smell affects the limbic region of the brain, which controls emotions, memory and the hypothalamus, which regulates the pituitary, which in turn balances the entire hormonal system of the body.

Art of the Apothecary

Apothecary is defined in today's terms as "a health professional trained in the art of preparing and dispensing drugs." Derived from the Greek word *apotheke*, it means a repository or store room and from the Hebrew word *raqach*, which means to perfume. Some bible translations use the word perfumer instead of apothecary, such as "to prepare spices." In biblical times, the Levitical priesthood served as apothecaries as well. One of the responsibilities for the priests included preparing the holy anointing oil and incense. In Exodus 30:22 - 28, we read about the instructions the LORD gave to Moses concerning the ingredients of the holy anointing oil:

"Moreover the LORD spake unto Moses, saying, Take thou also unto thee principal spices, of pure myrrh five hundred shekels, and of sweet cinnamon half so much, even two hundred and fifty shekels, and of sweet calamus two hundred and fifty shekels, And of cassia five hundred shekels, after the shekel of the sanctuary, and of oil olive an hin: And thou shalt make it an oil of holy ointment compound after the art of the apothecary: it shall be an holy anointing oil."

This highly perfumed formula prescribed by God comprised of the finest spices: flowing myrrh, sweet-smelling cinnamon, fragrant calamus cane, cassia and olive oil. Specific instructions for its use consecrated or set apart articles for Temple worship as "holy." This included the ark of the testimony, the holy tabernacle, and all of its furnishings. Because of its specialness, Yahweh gave an admonition to NOT reproduce the EXACT formula, nor use it on ordinary people. This is something believers should respect as they explore study and create biblical scents.

God not only gave Moses specific instructions for combining these essences for the Holy Anointing Oil, but for also combining them into a pure and Holy confection to be burned as an incense as a testimony in the tabernacle of the congregation before Yahweh. In Exodus 30:34 - 38, it says:

"And the LORD said unto Moses, Take unto thee sweet spices, stacte, and onycha, and galbanum; these sweet spices with pure frankincense: of each shall there be a like weight: And thou shalt make it a perfume, a confection after the art of the apothecary, tempered together, pure and holy: And thou shalt beat some of it very small, and put of it before the testimony in the tabernacle of the congregation, where I will meet with thee: it shall be unto you most holy. And as for the perfume which thou shalt make, ye shall not make to yourselves according to the composition thereof: it shall be unto thee holy for the LORD. Whosoever shall make like unto that, to smell thereto, shall even be cut off from his people."

Apothecaries remained a prominent part of Israel's culture after being taken into Babylonian captivity and upon returning to Jerusalem during the time of Nehemiah and Ezra. In Nehemiah 3:8 it tells how they participated in the rebuilding of the city:

"Next unto him repaired Uzziel the son of Harhaiah, of the goldsmiths. Next unto him also repaired Hananiah the son of one of the apothecaries, and they fortified Jerusalem unto the broad wall."

Though the term "apothecary" is not found in the New Testament, the practice of compounding and burning Holy Incense still continued. In fact, this duty was considered such a great honor for those of the Levitical priesthood they had to cast lots for it. Luke 1:9 tells how lot fell on Zacharias:

"According to the custom of the priest's office, his lot was to burn incense when he went into the temple of the Lord. And the whole multitude of the people were praying without at the time of incense. And there appeared unto him an angel of the Lord standing on the right side of the altar of incense."

Some may consider the duties of the apothecary and priest to be a lost art since the destruction of the 2nd Temple. However, Yeshua spoke of another temple (His body) in which believers are members of and are to be a priest unto. 1 Peter 2:5 says,

"Ye also, as lively stones, are built up a spiritual house, a holy priesthood, to offer up spiritual sacrifices, acceptable to God by Jesus Christ."

Today, the ancient art of perfumery and apothecary is being restored.

Methods of Making Perfume

Making perfume is an art that's been around for many centuries. To many, it's much more than an art. It's a creation of thought, inspiration and care, resulting in some of the most beautiful fragrances imaginable.

Although there have been different methods implemented through the years, the general principle and purpose of making perfume is the same: extracting a desired scent. In an earlier chapter we covered many methods of extracting fragrances from various plant parts. There are actually two methods of scent extraction today: effleurage or distillation.

• Effleurage is a process where a glass plates are filled with highly purified and odorless animal or vegetable fat, where petals of your choice are placed. The petals of fresh flowers are pressed into the fat and will stay in the grease for a few days so the essence has a chance to disperse and leak into the compound.

After a few days, the petals are removed and replaced with freshly picked ones. This process continues until the greasy compound is saturated with the essence. This process is repeated several times. Once the saturation point has been reached, the petals are removed and the grease and fragrant oil mixture, also known as effleurage pomade, is washed with alcohol so that extract can separated from the grease.

The remaining grease is used to make soap and, once the alcohol evaporates, you have the essential oil you need for perfume. Effleurage is not only very time consuming but an expensive way of extraction as well. This process is often used for Jasmine and tuberoses.

•   Distillation is a process where steam is used to capture the fragrance. The plants or flowers are put in the top part of a sill on perforated trays, with the bottom part filled with water. The water is brought to a boil, as it's the steam that brings out the fragrances and scent-bearing components, which are transferred into an attached glass-cooling worm to be refrigerated and condensed.

The essential oil and water mixture is placed in bottles, where the essential oils will rise to the top leaving the scented water on the bottom. While the scented water is used for toilette water and other purposes, the essential oil is made into the finest perfumes.

Although technology has provided perfume makers with state-of-the-art equipment to make their perfume quickly and efficiently, the methods are still basically the same. Once they have the desired perfume, they don't stop there. Being chemists as well as artists of the trade, they're able to mix them with other essential oils to create exotic and beautiful fragrances.

The Fragrant Makeup

Any perfume you buy or make yourself is a chemical compound made from fragrant oils, aroma blends, fixatives and solvents which produces a pleasant or attractive smell. Women primarily use perfume in order to smell nice for work, a special event, or even to attract a mate.

The composition of any perfume starts with base perfume oils, which are natural, animal or synthetic, and are then diluted with a solvent to make them light and applicable. Perfume oils in the purest form can cause damage to skin or an allergic reaction, so the adding of solvent is necessary to make them less potent. The most prevalent solvent used in the manufacturing of perfumes is Ethanol.

Plants are the oldest source for obtaining fragrant oil compounds from flowers and blossoms parts. Other plant parts, such as leaves, twigs, roots, rhizomes, bulbs, seeds, fruit, wood, bark and lichens are also considered for use in perfume making.

Perfumes made using animal sources are normally made from Musk, which is obtained from either the Asian Musk Deer or Civets (known as Civet Musk), as well as Ambergis (a fatty compound). Some perfume makers may also use either Castoreum or Honeycomb in the production of their perfumes.

Synthetic source perfumes are produced through organic synthesis of multiple chemical compounds, in which such things as Calone, Linalool, Coumarin and Terpenes are used to make synthetic fragrant oils. By using synthetic products in perfume making, you can produce scents which may not even exist in nature. In fact, this has become a very valuable element in the making of perfumes nowadays.

A perfume composition will either be used to augment other products, or patented and sold as a perfume after it has been allowed to age for one year.

Unfortunately, fragrance compounds will, after time, begin to deteriorate and lose strength if stored incorrectly. It is therefore important when making your own perfume that you store them in tightly sealed containers and keep them out of light and away from heat, as well as away from oxygen and other organic substances. For best results, store containers in a fridge at a temperature of between 33 and 40 degrees Fahrenheit.

Today more than ever, perfume is popular around the world, because of its use and its application continues to grow.

Steps to Perfume Making

If you carry out a search on the internet on "making perfume," you will find there is a wealth of knowledge on the many processes. You will find different recipes to experiment with, but the most important thing you should consider is what sort of perfumes you would like as your finished product.

First, you need to consider what sort of perfume you would like to make? Would it be an eau de cologne, perfume concentrate or even an aftershave?

Second, you need to decide what it should smell like? Do you want it to be soft or strong, sweet or manly or unisex? Does it have to be long lasting?

After answering these questions as to what kind of perfume you would like to make, you need to start making a list of the ingredients that you need. When making the list, think about the characteristics of the various ingredients you want to include in your recipe.

If you already have a recipe that you would like to use, it may mean you do not need to bother experimenting with the ingredients you have (it may be wise to adjust the quantities of the ingredients you are using in order to make the perfume more personalized). If you do not have your list of ingredients already prepared, there are a couple things that you should know prior to making your list.

When making perfume it is important that you experiment as much as you can. It should be remembered that perfume making is an art, and imagination and a great sense of smell will help you to overcome any lack of knowledge or experience.

The next most important thing in relation to perfume making is that there are 4 key ingredients you will need to produce perfume:

1. Essential Oils (these have been extracted from various plants (organic or non-organic) and when combined give the smell of the perfume you are trying to produce. The three different categories of oils include: Base notes, Middle notes, and Top notes. Each note ultimately influences the scent of your perfume over time. Perfume is seldom made with just one fragrance. They're usually a blend of up to three or more fragrances. This will be discussed in more detail in the next chapter.

2. Pure Grain Oil
If you plan to resell your perfume to the public, then you will need to use Perfumer's Alcohol (which can be hard to find locally, but available online) because the Department of Tobacco, Alcohol and Firearms does not allow selling products with Vodka in them. However, if you are only making your perfume for personal use, you can substitute 100-Proof Vodka in most recipes calling for Perfumers' Alcohol or Grain Alcohol.

Be sure to do a "skin patch test" to make sure you are not allergic to any of your ingredients by placing a drop on your skin and watching to see if a rash or irritation occurs. If so, discontinue use immediately.

3. Water
Use distilled water if any recipe calls for water. Never use tap water in its place.

4. Fixatives

Fixatives are used with the other ingredients in order to lower the rate of evaporation of the fragrance or essential oils. The reason why a perfume may lose its fragrance faster than normal is because only a little amount of fixative was used when preparing the perfume.

In some cases, you may want to use a vegetable oil in addition to a carrier oil with the essential oils. This will make up 10 to 35 percent of the finished perfume. Many perfumers recommend using Jojoba oil, as it has a long shelf life and is healthy for the skin. For those that don't know what Jojoba or a carrier oil is, it is to help dilute and blend your three fragrances together before they can be applied to your skin.

Understanding Notes

It's important when planning to make your own perfume to understand the basics. When we think of expensive perfume, we automatically think of France, since France is the perfume capital of the world. Although the French did not discover perfume, they were the ones that turned making perfume into a Science.

While the perfumers in France were not the original creators of perfume, they were the geniuses that figured out a way to make the fragrances last longer than just a few minutes. Their method of layering the different fragrances in three layers is what we now call "notes."

If you've never made perfume before, you may not know the importance of using the different notes. For the best fragrances, you can't just throw together several essential oils and hope for the best. Some fragrances are stronger and longer lasting than others. Knowing what essential oils are in each note group will help you to make some beautiful and interesting creations with your perfume. Notes are what make up the difference between perfume and cologne.

Perfumery is a science. Today's perfumes are mainly made with synthetic copies of essential oils as real oils would be too expensive to use in the mass production of perfume.

You will find most perfumes on the market today are diluted with alcohol and water. In your own laboratory, you may also want to use oil to dilute your perfume, although using alcohol will make them last longer. As you begin to blend your fragrances, you will want to experiment with a variety of different aromas. Most perfumes fall into one of the five categories:

Woodsy/Earthy: Cedarwood, Cypress, Pine, Patchouli, Vetiver, Myrrh and Sandalwood.

Floral/Oriental: Geranium, Jasmine, Neroli, Lavender, Rose and Ylang-Ylang

Herbal: Angelica, Basil, Chamomile, Clary Sage, Peppermint, and Rosemary.

Spicy: Black Pepper, Cardamom, Cinnamon, Clove, Coriander, Ginger, Neroli, Juniper, and Nutmeg.

Citrus: Bergamot, Grapefruit, Lemon, Lime, Mandarin, Orange, and Lemongrass

It will require a bit of experimentation with essential oils to get the scent that you want. Making perfume is definitely an art and, like any art, the result will depend on the time, inspiration and imagination that go in the product.

As stated earlier, perfume is seldom made with just one fragrance. They're usually a blend of up to three or more fragrances, consisting of base notes, middle notes and top notes.

Base notes, usually the backbone of the perfume, is what the users will remember most about this particular fragrance. This scent of base notes will last the longest in the air. Examples of base notes are Vanilla, Sandalwood, Lichens, Cinnamon, mosses or other woodsy scents. The middle notes are usually the inspiration for the perfume and often a floral scent such as Geranium, Honeysuckle, Jasmine, Lemongrass or Neroli. Top notes are usually the selling point for the perfume as well as the first name listed. Common top notes include Rose, Lavender, Orchid, Lemon, Bergamot or other citrus or herbal scents. In fact, Bergamot oil is one of the most widely essential oils used in the perfumery and toiletry industry, together with Neroli and Lavender, as the main ingredients for the classical Eau-de-cologne fragrance. These notes can also be followed by another ingredient to bridge the fragrances such as Peppermint, Chamomile, Marjoram, and Bay.

As with any good creation, it's combining the right mixture of ingredients that counts. Using notes that go well with each other will give you a beautiful fragrance you'll never tire of wearing. Your friends will constantly be asking you what you're wearing and where you got it. Imagine their surprise when you tell them it's your own creation!

One of the keys to successful perfume making is in mixing the right blend. Don't just assume because you happen to like two different fragrances that they'll make a good mixture for perfume. Before you waste a lot of time and money on essential oils, make some samples. Although making your own perfume is a lot cheaper than buying perfume, essential oil can get costly as well.

If you're considering blending a couple different oils together, put them on a cotton swap or perfume tester strip and let them sit overnight. In the morning, check out what they smell like. If you're pleased with the results, you have your new perfume fragrance and are ready to start creating your own masterpiece!

A. The Base Oil (Base Notes) – This will produce the scent that stays longest on the skin and for this reason it is usually added to the mixture first. Some of the fragrances with a base note include: Sandalwood, Vanilla, Patchouli, Cedarwood, Clove, Cinnamon, Mosses, Lichens, Ferns and Frankincense.

Base notes are what you smell after about 30 seconds of applying it to your skin. The base and middle notes are what make up the main fragrance of the perfume. However, for a perfume to be successful, they must have a combination of all three notes.

B. The Middle Oil (Middle Notes) – This also influences the smell of the perfume for quite some time, but not as long as the base notes does. Some of the fragrances with a middle note include: Lemongrass, Geranium, Rosewood, Neroli, Jasmine, Rose, Hyacinth and Ylang-Ylang.

Middle notes are what we smell when the scent from the top notes disappears. It is generally considered as the heart of the perfume and often server to cover up any unpleasant scents that may come from the base notes. This scent often evaporates after 15 seconds.

C. Top Oils (Top Notes) – This is added to the mixture after the middle notes, and may then be followed by some other substance which will help to bridge the scents together. Some of the fragrances that are top note include: Orchid, Rose, Bergamot, Chamomile, Lavender, Peppermint, Lemon, Orange and Lime.

Top notes are the scents that you smell as soon as you apply it. If you've ever sprayed a perfume in a store, the smell you get immediately after spraying is coming from the top notes. The top notes, although they quickly evaporate, are what gives us our first impression of a perfume.

Your fragrance will contain one or more from each of the above categories: base note, mid note and a top note. Some perfumers recommend using a four note, a bridge notes such as Lavender or Vanilla. The bridge is what will help the other three oils blend together and is often Vitamin

E oil, Jojoba oil or carrier oil, which you can get at a health food store.

The top note is the first to evaporate on your skin. It is also the first impression that you have of the fragrance. The mid note stays on a little bit more and the base note is what will remain on your skin for hours.

The base note will react with your skin to form a scent of its own. This is why no two perfumes smell exactly alike on any two people. It is also the reason why you should test out a perfume for about a half an hour by putting a dab on your wrist, do your shopping then taking a sniff to see if you still like the scent.

It is very important that when you are making perfume, you mix the extracts in the above order starting with base, then the middle and finally adding the top note. Typically, you can add equal amounts of each type in order to produce a quality perfume or follow the recommended basic formula in this book.

It takes a bit of trial and error when mixing blends at home. Perfumery is an art unto itself and takes years to practice. Perfumers today still practice this art and make scents that fail. It is all a matter of personal taste and seeing what blends well with what.

Perfumes were commonly used as aphrodisiacs to attract a mate. Today many perfumes are packaged and described as sensual. This term is used to describe its erotically-stimulating effect because of the components such as Musk or exotic blossom notes used in creating its fragrance. Such perfumes can produce pleasant emotions and moods, since the sense of smell is directly connected with the part of the brain in which feelings and sexual behavior are controlled.

Most of the perfume recipes in this book will require only a few drops worn at a time, by just dabbing on your wrists and behind your ears to carry the scent with you throughout the day. Because the essential oils are so concentrated in this blend, you do not want to use too much.

There is an old saying that your perfume should not walk in the room before you do. You want people to remember a pleasant scent, not be overpowered with fragrance.

You will find the recipes listed in this book also beneficial such as relaxing or for mental clarity. The benefits of using aromatherapy in your own perfumes are the following:

• Completely natural products and non-toxic

• Have healing powers as well as a pleasant fragrance

• Unique Scent (don't underestimate this one - there are people who pay plenty to create their own scent at perfumeries in Paris).

• Much less expensive in the long run

Keep in mind, when making your perfume, that you can mix and match different essential oils to get the scent that you want. The purpose of using the specific notes is to ensure you have a fragrance that's not only appealing but one that lasts as well.

When Buying Essential Oils

If you choose to use pure essential oils to make your perfumes, here are some helpful tips and suggestions on what to look for when buying essential oils.

You will want to look for 100% undiluted pure essential oils. If they're truly undiluted, you won't have to put your nose right up them to get a good whiff. You should be able to hold it about 5 inches away and still get a good smell. Another way to determine if they're undiluted is by putting a drop on a piece of paper. If it leaves an oily stain on the paper, it's probably been diluted with a vegetable oil.

Try not to smell too many in one day. Unbelievably, you nose will become overwhelmed and they'll all tend to smell the same.

Essential oils come in a variety of different prices, with some more expensive than others. If you find a store that offers them at the same price, this may be a sign they are synthetic.

One of the main reasons why you may not want to use synthetic oils is that they will not have the same therapeutic properties as true essential oils. Check the label to ensure it doesn't say perfume oil or fragrant oil.

The nice thing about using "therapeutic" perfumes that you make yourself is that the essential oils can actually help heal anything troubling you, or even give you energy, while also giving you a pleasant scent. Regular perfumes made with synthetics cannot boast of this power.

Avoid purchasing essential oils that have been stored in plastic bottles. Essential oils will dissolve the plastic causing it to become contaminated. Clear glass bottles are also not good for essential oils as they often make the oil spoil quicker. Look for essential oils that have been stored in dark bottles, particularly blue or dark amber.

If essential oils are very cheap in price, take a second look as they may not be pure essential oils. While they don't have to be 100% pure essential oils for perfume making, you'll get a much better and longer lasting scent with pure essential oils.

Making Your Own Fragrance

Have you ever put your two perfume bottles side by side and wished you could combine them? By making your own perfume, that's exactly what you can do. Here's a list of everything you'll need to begin the art of making your own perfume.

- Dark bottles for storing your perfume
- Three Fragrances or Essential oils
- Cotton swabs or perfume tester strips
- Glass droppers or pipettes (at least four)
- Jojoba oil or another carrier oil
- Plastic sheeting or newspaper to protect work space
- Labels for your bottles

Now that you have your favorite fragrances or notes, you're ready to get started. You are going to want to choose one fragrance from each category: top, base and middle. This will make a harmonious blend.

The following is a basic recipe for your perfume formula:

What You Will Need:
½ Ounce Jojoba Oil
2 ½ Ounce Alcohol
6 Drops Top Note Essential Oil
7 Drops Middle Note Essential Oil
7 Drops Base Note Essential Oil
Dark Bottle

What To Do:

1. Using a clean, dark glass bottle, add your base carrier oil such as Jojoba first.

2. When adding essential oils, start with the base note then add the middle note, followed by the top note. As you add each one, check the scent to make sure it is what you are looking for.

3. Add the alcohol then shake for several minutes. Allow your blend to sit for 48 hours up to six weeks. The longer it sits, the stronger the scent.

4. Store your perfume in a dark glass bottle. Don't forget to name your creation!

This basic recipe can be changed and adapted to your own signature style, depending on what you like. Keep track of what you add or change, so you'll know how to make your favorite blends at a later time.

You will have to play around with scents for a little bit before you hit on what you like. Make sure that you write each ratio of every essential oil used in a particular scent as nothing can be more frustrating than actually coming up with the fragrance of your dreams and then not remembering how you ended up making it.

Whether it's soft and subtle or exotic and romantic, you can easily make any fragrance you desire. The possibilities are endless. So, get ready to make the formation of a lifetime!

It is a good idea to do a test sample of the mixture you have chosen before actually making the perfume. From the fragrances you're considering, place a drop of each one on a cotton swab, and let it sit overnight. If it's what you want in the morning, you're all ready to start. One possible selection could be Sandalwood essential oil for the base,

Orchid essential oil for the top and Honeysuckle essential oil for the middle note.

Before you begin, cover your workspace with plastic or old newspaper as essential oils can easily stain your table or countertops. You'll want to use a separate pipette or dropper for each note you use.

The perfect combination blend consists of one part top, one part middle, two parts base and one part jojoba oil or other carrier oil. For instance, you'll use one part Honeysuckle, one part Orchid, one part Carrier oil and two parts Sandalwood. Keep in mind, each part may be up to 40 drops, depending on your container size.

Using a pipette, extract each essential oil into the bulb to place in your bottle. You may need to squeeze more than once to get the amount you want. Just make sure you use the right ratios. Remember to use a separate pipette or glass eye dropper for each of the oils used. You will not be adding the carrier oil at this time.

When you're essential oil blend is all mixed in the container, put a lid on the container and let them sit for at least a day or two in a cool, dark place. After sitting, the fragrance will intensify. Take the cover off and see if it has the desired scent you are looking for. If so, you're ready to add your carrier oil. If not, you can add more essential oils and let it sit longer until you get the desired scent. If you're satisfied, cover it tightly once again and let it sit. This time you may want to let it sit for at least a week so the fragrances can really get to work. At the end of this maturing process, you should have the perfume of your dreams!

Getting Your Desired Fragrance

Making your own perfume can provide you with a lot of fun while enabling you to make your own signature scents. Once you get the hang of what you're doing, you'll want to make several different scents for friends and family. These make very special gifts as the recipient will look at them as a personal gift you made just for them.

As mentioned earlier, perfume consists of three major components. These components are essential oils, distilled water and perfumer's alcohol or Vodka. While you have the option of experimenting with different fragrances and oils, it's important that you pay special attention to which oils you're using for each note: top, middle, and base.

For instance, the top note is going to be the first scent you smell when you apply the perfume. While it may be a great smelling fragrance, it usually disappears within 15 seconds and is replaced by the middle note. The middle note; however, disappears within 30 seconds to be replaced by the base note. In spite of these scents and how they seem to disappear, they all play a part in what your finished product will smell like and how long the scent will last.

Of particular importance is the order in which your notes are added because this will play a part in how they smell as the finished perfume as well as how long the scent will last. The base note should go in first, followed by the middle note and finally the top note goes in last.

One of the most important reasons for making your own perfume is to get a desired scent or fragrance. You may have a general idea of what you're looking for but aren't sure how to get it when choosing your essential oils. For instance, your husband likes cologne that has a woodsy scent.

Buying this in a store is easy because he'll be able to provide you with a name. However, when making your own perfume or cologne, you may not know how to achieve these desired scents.

When using pure essential oils, there will be quite a difference to ratios when making perfumes. These are meant to be used sparingly. For instance, you will dilute the perfume with one tablespoon of carrier oil or alcohol to about 30 drops of essential oils. As you can see, the ratio between essential oils and either carrier oil or alcohol is almost equal.

Therefore, to make things a little easier for you, I've listed some of the most popular scents and the essential oils you can use to achieve those scents or fragrances.

Floral scents are achieved by using Jasmine, Geranium, Ylang-Ylang, Rose or Neroli.

Herbal scents can be achieved by the use of Chamomile, Angelica, Rosemary, Basil, Peppermint, Lavender or Clary Sage.

For earthy scents, you can use Vetiver or Patchouli. For the woodsy scents so many men like, try using Cedarwood, Sandalwood, Pine or Cypress.

Spicy scents are easy to get with Cinnamon, Black Pepper, Ginger, Cardamom, Nutmeg, Clove, Juniper or Coriander.

Fruity scents can be achieved with Bergamot, Lime, Lemon, Orange, Grapefruit, Lemongrass or Mandarin.

The Art of Perfumery

Perfume making can be easy or complex depending on the bouquet of fragrances you choose.

As mentioned earlier, essential oils are the most common sources to use for your perfume making. The oils used will establish the perfume's inherent attributes, like mood, quality and character. Since they are concentrated oils, essential oils may seem costly for what you get, but they do go a long way. In fact, most perfumes require only a couple of drops of essential oil. You will be amazed at the many different fragrances you will find online or at any health food store. Some people that don't use essential oils due to their cost instead use food flavorings like orange, almond, vanilla, etc.

If you're really interested in cutting corners and being creative, you can also make perfume with lemon or orange peels that have been dried. Another choice is using dried flowers such as dry Rose petals or Lavender. Your choices are almost endless for what you can use for your fragrances. Once you've decided what fragrance or scent you want, you're all ready to begin the process.

For some beginners, you may want to start off with just one scent. After you get the hang of it, you can experiment with several scents but for now, using one scent will make it easier! You'll want to mix a few drops of essential oil in a small jar with a tight fitting lid.

Keep in mind the more oil you use, the stronger the scent is going to be. Add four tablespoons of both Vodka and distilled water. Mix well, cover tightly and let sit for at least a week. You may want to test sample your perfume occasionally by putting a cotton swab in the mixture and rubbing it on your skin. If it smells the right strength, you're done.

If you'd like a stronger scent, you can add a drop or two more of essential oil and let it sit for a few more days in a cool dark place. When it's ready to use, strain it through a coffee filter into a dark perfume bottle. The scent will stay longer if your store your perfume in a cool dark room. Keep in mind that if you use orange peels, it will take longer for the scent to become strong than if using essential oils.

One perfumer suggested, "The strength of the perfume is dependent upon the ratio of fragrant oils, alcohol and water in the blend. Each blend will smell different and the amount of essential oil is critical. A single drop too much, or too little, will change the characteristic of the perfume completely."

The art of making perfume is an art anyone can master. If you have the supplies and a little imagination, you'll find making perfume is fun and very easy. Whether it's something you want to tackle on your own or as a way to bond with your daughter, making perfume is a great way to spend an afternoon or evening. As easy as it is to make perfume, there are certain myths about making perfume or little hints that may help you to achieve the fragrance you desire.

Although one drop of an essential oil may not seem like very much, these oils are in their purest undiluted form. A few drops goes a long way, so unless you want a perfume that's overwhelming and overpowering, follow the directions carefully. If it says five drops, use five drops. It's much easier to add more drops if you desire a stronger scent than it is to remove drops when the perfume is too strong!

While we're on the subject of overwhelming perfumes, you may notice that your nose may not be working as
it usually does after you've smelled so many different
essential oils. In other words, what's actually a very strong
scent your nose may not be picking it up as such. There's a
very simple way to correct this problem. Hold coffee
grounds or fresh coffee beans a couple inches from your
nose and inhale several times. You'll soon find your nose
working once again!

To avoid making perfumes with weird and off-the-
wall fragrances, make sure you stay with a base, middle and
top note. As much as you may like many different fragrances, not all of them will go well together. It's also
imperative that you put in the oils in a specific order, which
is base, middle and top is last.

If someone tells you that you can use tap water instead of distilled water, don't listen to him or her. Using
distilled water is necessary for your perfume venture to be
successful. You can substitute Vodka instead of alcohol
though if you are reselling your perfume. In fact, Vodka
works excellently with perfume as it enhances the fragrance,
making it last longer. You may want to try brandy but keep
in mind that it will not blend well with all oil fragrances.

Again, don't forget to take notes while you're making
your perfume. It will serve not only for all of your successful
choices, but also for failures.

Hints That Make Scents

Here are some very helpful hints regarding making perfume. Keep these tips in mind while making your perfume, so things will go smoother and more economical.

• Before actually purchasing any essential oils, test them on your skin first to make sure you don't have a reaction to them.

• If you're considering blending a couple different oils together, put them on a cotton swab or perfume tester strip and let them sit overnight. In the morning, check out what they smell like and if you're pleased with the results, you are ready to start creating your own masterpiece!

• The higher the percentage of essential oils you use, the stronger your perfume is going to be. Typical ratios percentages are 70 to 85 percent alcohol, 5 percent water and 15 to 30 percent essential oils.

• Do NOT substitute tap water for spring or distilled water.

• When using Vodka, make sure you use 100-proof Vodka.

• If you want some color in your perfume, add a natural, good grade vegetable food dye.

• When making your perfume, be sure to take notes so if it's a success, you'll know exactly what you did so you can do it again.

• Your perfume will last must longer if you store it in a dark bottle. It should also be stored in a glass container as opposed to plastic.

• When adding the essential oils to your perfume mixture, use separate eyedroppers for each essential oil to avoid contamination or spoiling the fragrance of your perfume. If you don't have enough eyedroppers, make sure to wash them thoroughly after each use. Try washing them in alcohol or Vodka to clean thoroughly.

• Remember to use base notes, middle notes and top notes when making your perfume. Make sure to add them in proper order and use the right oils for specific notes. As stated earlier, typical top notes are Bergamot, Lemon, Neroli or Lavender while base notes are Cinnamon, Cedarwood, Sandalwood or Vanilla and middle notes are Lemongrass, Geranium, Clove, and Neroli or Ylang-Ylang.

• When your perfumes are in the curing stage, keep in mind the longer they sit before use, the stronger they'll be and the longer the scent will last.

• Don't be afraid to experiment. You may be surprised at some of the luxurious scents you can make with a little experimentation.

• After practicing on perfume-making, try making your own body sprays, solid perfume and even men's cologne at home.

• Essential oils can become costly, especially if you are planning to make a combination of many scents. However, if you know you'll be doing this more than once, you can often save money by buying a "package deal" of several oils. Keep in mind; however, that even a small container of essential oils goes a long way.

• If you're not sure of which scents you are going to want to use, take advantage of the samples that are offered in many health stores. Often by taking a sniff or two, you'll have a better idea of which ones you want to buy.

• When making any homemade perfume, it is important that you use the right materials for not just measuring, but for handling, mixing and storing the finished product in.

• Do not use utensils you already have in your kitchen (ones for measuring water or food items), as they are not suitable for measuring fragrance oils, alcohol and other such solutions that are required to make perfume. It is better that you use measuring devices that allow you to exactly measure out the amounts of oils and solvents required. If you do not, the perfume you make may not be what you wanted. It is best if you use measuring devices made from glass so that you can see what is inside. When handling any formulas (i.e., transferring them to storage bottles or other containers), use a funnel with a narrow long neck.

• When making solid perfume, an empty and cleaned Chapstick tube makes a great container for storage. It's also easy to apply with this tube.

• Subtle scents of solid perfume smell great on your business cards when used in moderation.

• Scents that have a citrus or woodsy aroma are perfect for use in making men's cologne. They're not too powerful yet their scent lasts for hours. In fact, citrus oils will usually keep their scents for up to six months.

• Consider making perfumes with scents that are more than just for "decoration" or smell. Cedarwood essential oil makes a great-smelling perfume that is effective for repelling insects; while Ginger or Orange essential oils are perfect for providing your body with a warming sensation, particularly when used in solid perfumes. Check out my book, *Heal With Oil* or *Heal With Essential Oil: Nature's Medicine Cabinet* to learn about the many psychological effects of different scents such as Lavender for relaxation and calmness.

Simple Perfume Recipes

Before we get started, make sure you have everything you need. Here's your checklist.

- Distilled water
- Essential oils
- Plastic sheeting
- Glycerin
- Large measuring cup with spout for pouring
- Dark glass bottle with lid
- Vodka or Perfumer's Alcohol

You're probably still wondering about the Vodka, right? Using Vodka in your perfume will actually serve a couple of purposes. Vodka enhances the aroma of perfumes. It also preserves the scent without making it overpowering. You only need a small amount so don't rush out and buy a fifth!

The plastic sheeting is used to protect your table or countertop as the essential oils and alcohol can damage them if spilled. This is also the reason you're using a measuring cup with a spout. It's much easier to pour without worrying about spilling it. It's better to be safe than sorry.

When making homemade perfumes as previously discussed, there are four main ingredients which you will need, and these are:

1. Essential Oils
2. Water
3. Alcohol
4. Fixatives

Many of these items can be either obtained from a store that specializes in such ingredients, or over the internet.

You will also need a large saucepan, large bowl (for mixing all the ingredients together), spoon and some measuring cups or jugs to make perfume at home.

Provided below, are a few easy recipes that you should be able to produce at home without too much effort.

1. Basic Recipe
This first recipe uses flowers right in your backyard. All you need for this recipe is some water and chopped flower blossoms (use Lilac or Lavender essential oil if blossoms are unavailable).

If you like a floral scent, you'll love this simple perfume recipe. To start out, you'll need one to two cups of fresh flowers, petals or chopped blossoms (Roses, Lilacs, Carnations, etc.) and two cups of water. Get a medium size bowl and put cheesecloth on top, making sure it hangs over the side of the bowl.

Place one cup of your flower blossoms in the cheesecloth and cover them completely with water. The mixture needs to sit covered overnight. The next day lift the cheesecloth up and squeeze the cheesecloth over the saucepan so you'll get the scented liquid. Simmer this liquid until only about a teaspoon remains. Let it cool and pour it into a small dark bottle. Spray in the air as a freshener or use on the skin.

2. Basic Recipe #2
Place 25 drops of your favorite essential oils into your measuring cup. You may choose one or more fragrances to give you a compelling and deep fragrance but be sure to use fragrances that will go well with each other.

Add five drops of glycerin to the essential oils. Glycerin is used as a fixative because it will help your perfume keep its aroma much longer. Mix the glycerin and add 3 tablespoons of Vodka and 2 cups of distilled water. Stir the mixture with a spoon so that it's blended well. Now is when you want to check out the aroma to determine if it's strong enough for you. If not, add a drop or two until you have the exact strength you want. The longer you let your perfume sit, the stronger it will be as well, like fine wine! Your ratio should be 70 percent alcohol, 20 percent essential oils and 10 percent water.

Once you have the strength the way you like it and it's mixed well, pour your perfume into the dark glass bottles, making sure the lids are tight. Store it a cool dry location, letting it sit one full day before using.

3. Amazement
For this blend, you will need one cup of distilled water, five teaspoons of Vodka, and five drops each of the following essential oils: St. John's Wort, Cypress and Rosemary. They should then be mixed together and stored overnight.

After a period of 12 hours or more, the solution produced can be put into a dark spray bottle to be used. Using a dark colored bottle will help the solution to remain fresh, which will be felt by the person using it when they apply it to their skin.

4. Whispering Rain
This recipe breathes a light scent reminiscent of a lingering shower. Again, you will need one cup of distilled water, five teaspoons of Vodka, five drops of each: Sandalwood, Bergamot and Cassia essential oils (which can also be purchased as fragrance oils).

These ingredients should be stirred together and then stored overnight in a covered container. Then, the next day, it can be transferred to a dark colored bottle. This perfume must be kept in a cool place so that it does not dry up.

The three perfumes above normally last for about a month before they lose their scent. The next recipe should produce something a bit better.

5. English Country Garden

For this recipe, you will need five drops each of the following essential oils: Valerian, Chamomile, and Lavender. Add five teaspoons of Vodka and one cup of distilled water. All these ingredients should be put into a jar and then shaken. It should then be put in a cool place and left for a week. After this time, you can then transfer the mixture into small perfume bottles.

It is important to remember that these types of perfume recipes only have a shelf life of a month; therefore you will need to make new batches every few weeks.

6. Oriental

To bring a touch of the orient into your home, try mixing up this next recipe. Add four drops of Sandalwood, four drops of Musk, three drops of Frankincense essential oil and two drops of Jojoba oil into a small dark bottle with a tight fitting lid. Make sure you shake well after adding each essential oil is added to the bottle. Do not add everything to the bottle at one time and then shake it up. Store your blend in a dark place for at least 12 hours before using. The longer you let it sit, the stronger and longer lasting the scent will become.

This last recipe will make a delightful body splash with a citrus aroma.

7. Citrus Twist

You'll need two cups of distilled water, three table-spoons 100-proof Vodka, five drops of Lemon Verbena essential oil, ten drops of both Mandarin and Orange essential oils and one tablespoon each of finely chopped orange and lemon peel.

Add the orange and lemon peels to the Vodka and store in a covered jar for one week. When the week is over, pour the liquid through a strainer. Drop the essential oils in one at a time to the liquid, followed by the distilled water. Make sure you shake thoroughly after each addition before adding the next one. Cover again and let sit for two weeks, making sure to shake the mixture at least once each day. Once it's done, store the dark glass bottle in a cool dark place.

Invent Your Signature Fragrance

Using essential oils to make your own perfume is not only great fun, but also extremely satisfying as well. These natural perfumes can help to enhance a person's good mood, drive away a bad one, and help them to relax or even to provide them with some energy. It may even make you feel glamorous, exotic, confident or utterly feminine as well.

The recipes provided in this book are simple to make and easy to follow. All you need to do is choose which one you want to try. You may also want to do a search on the internet to see which essential oils blend well together and try them instead.

Follow these simple instructions provided below, to create your very own aromatherapy perfume.

First, you need a base. It can either be alcohol or a carrier oil (but the best is a mixture of the two together). The best type of alcohol to use is one which is odorless (Vodka) and mixes well with Jojoba. Jojoba is particularly good, as it has a long shelf life, and once it is put on the skin, it tends to dry out and leave a wonderful scent behind.

However, Jojoba is one of the more expensive carrier oils, and I would suggest you experiment with one of the cheaper ones (such as Almond or Apricot Kernel oil) until you are comfortable. Then, once you are happy with the product you've produced, you can make the same product but, using Jojoba oil instead.

The equipment you will need for making aromatherapy perfume is as follows:

• Measuring Spoons (Any kitchen store or department store will have these)

• Small Funnel (Can be purchased at any craft or kitchen store)

• Small Colored Bottles (Look around your local craft stores or search on the internet)

• Dropper (sometimes you can purchase dropper tops with essential oil bottles)

Popularity of Making Perfume

Just what is it about making perfume that makes it so popular? As mentioned earlier, recent studies on women wearing perfume, most of the women stated that they bought a particular scent perfume because it made them smell good, they felt more feminine and better about themselves. In short, they stated when they felt better about themselves, they felt more attractive.

This is one major reason why many women choose to make their own perfume. They know what they like and what makes them feel good but often can't find it in the store or can't afford the high price. Making your own perfume is very affordable!

As a gift, it can't more personal, special or unique than when you give some a bottle of perfume you've made specifically for them. With crafts and do it yourself projects so popular today, you can find almost any supplies you need for almost any project, including making perfume.

You'll have a lot of fun shopping for perfume bottles to store your unique creation. Thrift stores, garage sales and swap meets are great places to find vintage bottles, which add a great touch to your homemade perfume.

Many that have been making their own perfume for a long time and have it down to an art are doing it now for money. Research has shown once you know what you're doing; you can easily make up to 100 bottles of your favorite perfume for less than $300 dollars. That's only three dollars a bottle. If you sold each bottle for ten dollars, you'll have more than tripled your investment and the buyer is getting an excellent deal as well. It's a win-win situation for both parties!

There is another reason why many people are choosing to make their own perfume or cologne. Pure essential oils, which are in most perfumes, have many healing and holistic properties such as promoting relaxation, relieving stress, etc. By making their own perfume with essential oils, they're getting the best of both worlds. They smell great and are healthier for your body or for your family member's bodies. Consider the choices and reasons and you may soon join the many that are making their own perfume!

Learning Ingredient Benefits

You may have questions about different ingredients and what their purposes are in perfumes as well as what properties different scents can offer you. You may be amazed to learn that there may be a connection to the relaxing and calm feeling you have at certain times. It may be related to the scent of perfume you're wearing!

To make perfume that's well blended with the best possible fragrance, try to use a formula that consists of 15 to 30 percent essential oils, 70 to 85 percent alcohol or Vodka and at least 5 percent distilled water. These percentages can be adjusted according to your personal preferences.

Perfumer's alcohol works very well as carrier oil when making perfume. While many people use pure alcohol or some other carrier oil, high-quality Vodka works as a substitute because it's odorless and will enhance the fragrance and keep the scent alive longer. However, it should be noted that using Vodka makes a nice toilette water or linen spray, but will not match professional quality perfume. Perfume has at least 15% aromatic materials, usually higher. Using Vodka, you can only achieve around 5%, sometimes less with denser oils. Because of this, you may experience the Vodka and essential oil separating. This is because Vodka is made up of 40% Ethanol and the rest water. Ethanol, of course, is what dissolves the oily fragrance. The oils will separate from the Vodka if you go over a certain low percentage, which varies depending on the density. Hence, you will never be able to get a full-strength perfume from Vodka and essential oils. However, for the sake of creating perfumes for personal use at home, Vodka will suffice.

Essential Oils that come from the skins of many citrus fruits make the perfect top note for perfume. The invigorating scents they provide are not overpowering and are often appropriate for men's cologne as well as women's perfume. Other oils that work well for men's colognes are Verbena, Cypress and Lemongrass essential oils. All three of these oils will provide a slightly woodsy scent that men love and women find very appealing!

Jojoba oil is another excellent choice for a carrier oil or base. It's actually a liquid plant wax made from the Jojoba seeds. This non-greasy oil is easily absorbed and has a very long shelf life, making it a great buy.

Ylang-Ylang essential oil is a very popular fragrance in perfumes. Not only is it good as a base, but it's a popular choice for its calming and relaxing properties. Because it is considered one of the most erotic scents in the world, it's often used as an aphrodisiac. It works great for relaxing the muscles and calming the nerves.

Geranium essential oil is a delicate and rosy fragrance that's used often to treat stress and anxiety and to reduce fatigue. While it's very similar in properties to genuine Rose essential oil, it is much less expensive. It's known for bringing balance and harmony.

Patchouli essential oil is a warm and earthy fragrance that's an excellent choice for a women's perfume or a man's cologne. It's often used as a fixative because it will not evaporate quickly like some oils and will prolong the fragrance in your perfume.

In the same way that many health foods are used for natural and holistic healing, perfumes are also now being recognized for the many benefits they can provide the body. By learning more about that many available essential oils and their benefits, you'll be able to serve more than one purpose when making your own perfume.

Perfumes for Holistic Healing

With so many people switching to holistic or natural healing methods, essential oils are quite popular in helping us get back to the basics.

Did you know that certain scents and fragrances can alter your mood?

One of the things that make perfume making so much fun is being able to experiment with different essential oils until you get your favorite scent down to a science. By mixing up different essential oils, you may be able to alter your moods and senses.

In an article entitled, "Essential Oils for Mental and Emotional Health" written by Gayle Eversole, DHom, PhD, MH, NP, ND, she states, "The psycho-physiological effect essential oils can be observed with EEG. Cortical activity is altered in alpha, beta, delta, and theta waves. Research in Japan established that Jasmine oil increases alertness and attention through beta-wave activity. Jasmine oil can also offer a stimulating effect.

Scent has a special impact on living organisms. Scientific research into the human sense of smell finds it to be 10,000 times more powerful than taste. Scent travels rapidly to the brain, and is shown to have a direct effect on the limbic system. The limbic system communicates with the autonomic nervous system. This is the known connection in the brain to the hypothalamus, emotion, memory, and some visceral (gut) reactions. Since the 1980's olfactory research has promoted the psychological benefit of essential oils used in aromatherapy.

The central nervous system has much to gain with the use of essential oils. They can be anti-depressant, sedative, tranquilizing, and release endorphins. The hypothalamic response affects the endocrine system through hormone release. Ultimately, all cells in a living organism are touched through the use of the essential oils."

Here is a list of some very common essential oils as well as their properties or characteristics. After reading this, you're going to want to rush out, buy some of these essential oils and check their effectiveness!

Certain essential oils, for example, offer different psychological effects:

Anti-Depressant:
• Ylang-Ylang
• Geranium
• Jasmine
• Orange
• Sandalwood
• Lemon
• Lemon Verbena
• Mandarin

Anxiety:
• Petitgrain
• Neroli
• Bergamot
• Cypress
• Lavender
• Lime
• Marjoram
• Rose
• Violet Leaf

Innervating:
• Basil
• Peppermint
• Rosemary (Rosemary shows a positive effect in Alzheimer's)

Sedative:
• Neroli
• Petitgrain
• Cedarwood
• Chamomile
• Melissa
• Valerian

In addition to these, Grapefruit and Sandalwood essential oils can help to fight fear. Ylang-Ylang and Orange essential oils will help with anger. Lavender and Jasmine essential oils can help you relieve anxiety as well as help you sleep. Lavender essential oil is also great for skin problems and burns. That is why Lavender is called the universal essential oil. One of its many uses includes relaxation. Rosemary and Cypress essential oils can help build your confidence. Rosemary is also good for fatigue. Rose, Frankincense and Bergamot essential oils can help you deal with grief and depression.

Peppermint and Pepper essential oils are good for increasing your memory power. Peppermint essential oil is also good for clearing the mind and relief of headaches and migraines. It's also great for digestion discomfort. Lemon essential oil is calming, soothing and almost uplifting affect on the spirit and mind as well as fighting fatigue. Juniper, Sandalwood, Neroli and Cedarwood essential oils are good for lifting your spirits. Marjoram and Helichrysum essential oils work well to help fight panic.

While you may wonder how these essential oils can make a difference in your mood and spirits, many people have used them successfully for hundreds of years. If you're considering making your own perfume, why not try some of them? In addition to any healing effects they may have on your body, you may also find you've discovered some great new fragrances to wear.

Studies dating from the 1920s report the following benefits of selected essential oils:

- **Lavender:** relaxing, circulation, meditative.
- **Pine:** strengthening, stabilizing.
- **Angelica:** anorexia, relieving hopelessness.
- **Basil:** fatigue, general nerve tonic, anti-depressant, soporific, confusion, melancholy, mental clarity and concentration, reduces anxiety. (careful use prevents over-stimulation).
- **Bay:** anti-hysteric, sedative, hypotensive.
- **Bergamot:** sedative for anxiety and antidepressant, stimulates appetite.
- **Chamomile (Roman):** calming, hyperactivity, good for use with children.
- **Clary Sage:** sedative and nervine for insomnia, paranoia, panic, and hysteria.
- **Cypress:** anxiety, confusion.
- **Everlasting:** grounding, increases dream activity.
- **Juniper:** apathy, paranoia, confusion, anxiety, nervous trembling and paralysis, diuretic.
- **Marjoram:** grief, insomnia.
- **Spikenard:** grounding.

Perfumes Oils and Colognes

Now that you are familiar with creating fragrances using an alcohol base, in this chapter we will look at recipes for colognes and perfume oils. Perfumer, J. Michelle explains in her E-how article on perfume making that "In perfumery, alcohol is used as a preservative and to help disperse the scent. As the alcohol evaporates it sends molecules of the scent into the air. It is possible, and perfectly acceptable, to make perfume without alcohol by using a carrier oil instead. A carrier oil is any vegetable-based oil into which you blend your essential oils and other fragrances. Because they don't disperse as easily, perfume oils tend to linger on the skin longer, and smell stronger than alcohol-based perfumes."

The following recipes are all easy to make. Each recipe includes either essential or fragrance oils as part of the formula. The first will bring the scent of the Far East to you.

Far East Oil
4 Drops Sandalwood Essential Oil
4 Drops Musk Essential Oil
3 Drops Frankincense Essential Oil
2 Teaspoons Jojoba oil (carrier oil)

Mix all of the ingredients together in a bottle and shake well. Place them in a dark colored bottle then allow the perfume to settle for at least 12 hours. Once it has sat for 12 hours or more, you should now store it in a cool dry area.

As you can see making your own perfumes, colognes or body oils is simple. Once you've made your first lot and tried it yourself, you will soon want to be making more. Here are some more recipes for you to try at home.

Orient Perfume Oil

This pleasant oil works to promote energy as well as aid you in creating a romantic mood. Both Jasmine and Ylang-Ylang are powerful aphrodisiacs, so only use this blend with caution.

What You Will Need:

1 Tablespoon Carrier oil
15 Drops Sandalwood Essential Oil
5 Drops Jasmine Essential Oil
4 Drops Ylang-Ylang Essential Oil
Glass Bottle

What To Do:

1. Add your carrier oil to your bottle, followed by the essential oils in order by notes. Let stand overnight.

2. Shake bottle each day before use. Keep in mind, the longer it sits, the stronger the fragrance will be.

3. Test to see if it is your desired strength. If not, add a few drops of carrier oil to dilute, or more essential oil to strengthen its fragrance.

Sleep Tonight Fragrant Oil

Here's a simple recipe for a perfume guaranteed to help you sleep better at night. In this recipe, Lavender essential oil is going to be the top note and added last.

What You Will Need:

1 Teaspoon Perfumer's Alcohol or Vodka
1 Teaspoon Jojoba Oil
4 Drops Lavender Essential Oil
3 Drops Chamomile Essential Oil
2 Drops Marjoram Essential Oil
2 Drops Bergamot Essential Oil
Funnel
Dropper

What To Do:

1. Add one teaspoon of each: Perfumer's Alcohol and Jojoba oil in a bottle, using a funnel to avoid spilling and wasting any.

2. Using a dropper or pipette, add Chamomile, Marjoram, Bergamot and Lavender essential oils. Be sure to put the lid on the bottle after adding each essential oil, shaking well before adding the next.

3. After shaking well, store in a cool dark place for up to twelve days, making sure the lid is on tight. Each day the bottle should be shaken a couple of times to make sure the oils are mixed.

4. Place a dab on pulse points before bed, for a great night's sleep.

Sunshine Cologne

This recipe is not a perfume but cologne and contains Lemon as the main ingredient.

What You Will Need:
1 Cup Distilled Water
1 Cup Vodka or Perfumer's Alcohol
3 Drops Lemongrass Essential Oil
10 Drops Lavender Essential Oil
10 Drops Lime Essential Oil

What To Do:

1. Add the Vodka or perfumer's alcohol in the bottle first. Add the essential oils next in the order of each note and shake well. Set aside for three weeks.

2. After 3 weeks, you will need to add the distilled water and then let it stand for a further week. It is important that you shake the bottle once a day while it is matures over the four-week period.

3. After a month, transfer the mixture to dark bottles for storage, or keep the mixture in the bottle it is in, in a dark cool place.

Zesty Lime Cologne

This fragrance is refreshing and gives you energy. Lime is known for its benefits in skin care for oily and inflamed skin.

What You Will Need:
1 Cup Vodka or Perfumer's Alcohol
1 Cup Distilled Water
10 Drops Lime Essential Oil
10 Drops Lavender Essential Oil
3 Drops Lemongrass Essential Oil
Glass Bottle

What To Do:

1. Pour the Vodka in a glass bottle then add essential oils in the order of their note.

2. Shake to mix. Allow to sit for two to three weeks to mature.

3. Add distilled water then shake. Let the perfume sit for another week in a dark, cool place. Be sure to shake once a day.

4. Wear on pulse points to enjoy its zesty fragrance.

Wake Up Aftershave

This aftershave cologne will give him that extra boost of energy in the morning.

What You Will Need:
2 Cups Witch Hazel
2 Ounces Rose Water
2 Ounces Aloe Vera Gel
½ Ounce Glycerin
1 Drop Peppermint Essential Oil
1 Drop Eucalyptus Essential Oil
Spray Bottle

What To Do:

1. Add witch hazel, Rosewater, Aloe Vera Gel and Glycerin to the bottle first. Shake to mix.

2. Add essential oils in order by their note and shake to mix. To use aftershave, spritz on skin after shaving. This recipe makes 2 ½ cups.

Citrus Splash Aftershave

Have him splash this one on after his morning shave. Its mild antiseptic properties will help protect the skin and curb any razor burns.

What You Will Need:
5 Tablespoons Orange Floral Water
5 Tablespoons Apple Cider Vinegar
3 Tablespoons Witch Hazel
18 Drops Bergamot Essential Oil
18 Drops Lemon Essential Oil
6 Drops Neroli Essential Oil
Glass Bottle

What To Do:

1. Add floral water, vinegar and witch hazel to a clean glass bottle. Shake to mix.

2. Add essential oils in order of each note: base, middle, and top, shaking well after adding each one.

3. Set bottle aside for several days to mature, shaking each day. Store your bottle in a dark, cool place.

4. Shake cologne before each use. Dab a little on after shaving.

Surrender Cologne

Let go of your worries and cares of the world. This cologne not only smells good, but it helps combat stress and fatigue.

What You Will Need:
½ Pint Vodka or Perfumer's Alcohol
1 Cup Distilled Water
3 Drops Cedarwood Essential Oil
3 Drops Bergamot Essential Oil
2 Drops Frankincense Essential Oil
Glass Bottle

What To Do:

1. In a bottle, add the Vodka followed by the essential oils in their correct order according each note. Shake well then sit aside for three weeks.

2. Add distilled water then allow the perfume to cure for another week. Be sure to shake once a day.

3. To use, dab on pulse points to wear as cologne. For peaceful sleep, try placing a few drops on your pillow before bed.

Perfume Body Sprays

Is there anything quite as refreshing and relaxing as a nice hot shower? Stepping out of the shower can be even more refreshing when you have a beautifully fragrant bottle of body spray to spritz on. Whether you want the body spray for yourself or to give as gifts, you can easily make your own body spray in much the same way as if you were making perfume.

Mix your choice of fragrance or essential oils in a medium size bowl. You'll want to use three to four fragrances so you'll have your base note, middle note and top note. The reason for this is because not all scents blend and while some will give you the most powerful scent, others will add longevity to the fragrance. They each have their purpose but will need to be added in their specific order.

The base, which typically can be Cedarwood, Cinnamon or Sandalwood, will be the first oil added to the bowl. This will be your strongest scent and one that lasts the longest. The middle note, typically Geranium, Neroli, Clove or Ylang-Ylang, will last awhile but not as long as the base and is added after the base. The top note, which may be Lime, Lavender, Rose, Bergamot, Jasmine or Rose, is the last oil to add to the bowl. Also, this scent will be the strongest when you spray it on your skin. Use a total of approximately 35 drops of oil and mix well with a stir stick or straw.

In a container with a tight-fitting lid, add three teaspoons of pure alcohol, Perfumer's Alcohol or Vodka. This will help to enhance the fragrances as well as make the scents last longer. Add the oil mixture to the alcohol or Vodka, cover and shake thoroughly, making sure it's all blended.

The reason for shaking it thoroughly is so the scent of the alcohol is covered up with the fragrant scents and so the different oils get mixed together.

Add four ounces of white vinegar and two cups of distilled water to the mixture, again shaking well after each addition. Pour the complete mixture into a bowl, using a coffee filter to strain it and get rid of any impurities or sediments from the oil. Using a funnel to avoid spills, pour your perfumed body spray into small spray bottles. Shake before using and store in a cool dry place away from extreme heat and direct sunlight. Once you find how easy it is to make your own body spray, don't hesitate experimenting with different fragrances and oils.

In the next few pages you will find other recipes for creating your own perfume body sprays. These zesty natural sprays will refresh you and are great for taking on vacation or somewhere exotic. You will find these formulas simple to make and easy to follow.

Soothing Summer Body Spray

Cool off this summer with a body spray made with real cucumbers.

What You Will Need:
1 Cup Distilled Water
1 Tablespoon Witch Hazel
1 Teaspoon Lemon Essential Oil
1 Teaspoon Cucumber Oil or fresh peelings
Spray Bottle

What To Do:

1. Add all of the ingredients in a bottle and shake well to blend.

2. Allow mixture to sit overnight. Store your spritzer in the refrigerator until ready to use. Spray on body to cool down after a day in the sun.

Citrus Fruit Splash

Filled to the brim with real fruit extracts, this nourishing skin drink will moisturize your skin.

What You Will Need:
2 Cups Distilled Water
3 Tablespoons White Wine Vinegar
3 Tablespoons Vodka or Perfumer's Alcohol
1 Tablespoon Lemon Peel, finely chopped
1 Tablespoon Orange Peel, finely chopped
10 Drops Mandarin Essential Oil
10 Drops Orange Essential Oil
5 Drops Lemon Essential Oil
5 Drops Grapefruit Essential Oil
Glass Jar with Top or Stopper
Glass Bottle

What To Do:

1. Place the Orange and Lemon peels and Vodka in a glass jar and cover with a lid or stopper for one week.

2. Press the mixture through a sieve to extract all liquid.

3. Pour the liquid into the glass bottle. Add essential oils in order according to each note then add the vinegar and water.

4. Let the perfume stand for two weeks, shaking often. Store your body splash in a cool, dark place.

Citrus Spray

The final recipe provided below is one which will produce a body splash, rather than a perfume, and has a citrus aroma to it.

What You Will Need:
2 Cups Distilled Water
3 Tablespoons Vodka
1 Tablespoon Lemon &Orange Peel (finely chopped)
5 Drops Lemon Verbena Essential Oil
10 Drops Mandarin Essential Oil
10 Drops Orange Essential Oil

What To Do:

1. Mix the fruit peels with the Vodka in a jar, cover and let it stand for one week.

2. After the week, strain the liquid and add the essential oils in order according to each note and the distilled water to it.

3. Now let the mixture sit for a further two weeks, making sure you shake the jar well once a day during this time.

4. Place the final solution after the two weeks in a dark bottle(s), or keep it in a cool dark area.

Perfume for Your Dog

When we think of perfume or making perfume, what usually comes to mind is making a beautifully fragrant scent for a night on the town or a relaxing scent to spray on us after a long soak in the tub. What usually doesn't come to mind is making perfume for our dogs! However, it's very easy to make perfume for your dog.

Not only will your dog smell great but also the perfume I'm about to show you will also help repel ticks. Every year, hundreds of dollars is spent by dog owners on insect repellent when, for a much lower cost, their dog could be wearing great-smelling perfume and repelling those nasty insects in a holistic way.

Before we get started, make sure you have the following things, which can be purchases at a health food store, ready. If you have more than one dog, you can double or triple the recipe.

- Straw
- Mixing Bowl
- Container for dog's perfume
- Saucepan
- Water
- 7 Drops of Cedarwood Essential Oil
- 7 Drops of Citronella Essential Oil
- 6 Drops of Lemongrass Essential Oil
- 1 Tablespoon of Vitamin E
- 1 tablespoon of Beeswax

In your mixing bowl, add the beeswax first, followed by the vitamin E. Add a small amount of water in your saucepan and put it on the stove. Place the mixing bowl with the beeswax and vitamin E in the saucepan. Keep it on high heat until the water boils and the mixture melts completely. A double boiler may also work for this is you have one. You may want to wear gloves as this mixture gets extremely hot.

Take the saucepan off the stove and remove the mixing bowl. Add the essential oils to your mixture according to each note, one drop at a time, stirring it with a straw. You'll want to stir it quickly so it is all mixed before the wax starts to get hard again.

Quickly, while it's still in liquid form, pour the mixture into the container you plan to store it in. Allow at least 30 minutes for your dog's perfume to harden before use. Once hard, you can rub it on your dog's collar and enjoy how great your dog smells, while no longer being bothered by ticks!

Perfumes Your Kids Can Make

Have you been looking for a project to do with your child that's fun and easy? Making perfume is something that many people are now experimenting with for several reasons. With the high cost of perfume in stores, many prefer to make it themselves, saving money as well as allowing them to make their own signature scent.

From the time girls are little, they love playing with and wearing perfume, whether it's toy perfume or their mother's best perfume. Making perfume is a project you can do with your daughter, niece, granddaughter or any young girl you know that likes having fun. Included here are three very simple recipes that even a young girl can understand and help with. They will find them so much fun, they'll want to take them to school to show their class!

Simple Bouquet

Find some spices and flowers that you enjoy smelling like Rosemary, Roses, Lavender, etc. Pick as many as you can so you'll have a stronger scent.

Place them in a saucepan or bowl and finely grind them with a mortar and pestle. Add a little water to the mixture. You may also want to try a blender for the grinding, making sure to add some water. Add some pure alcohol to the ground up mixture.

Pour your mixture through a strainer so you'll have all liquid. Pour the liquid either in a spray bottle or a used perfume bottle. Your little ones will love this!

Although this perfume won't be done for at least a week, it's still fun to make, particularly if you live with the little girl so she can smell the progress each day.

Recipe #2

Collect some flowers or plants that you both enjoy smelling. Encourage her to pick her favorites, whether they're Roses, Carnations or Daisies or anything from your herb garden. Find a jar with a tight fitting lid and fill it up with odorless oil. Cut the flowers off the stems and immediately put them in the jar containing the oil and close the lid tightly. It's most effective if all the flowers fall into the oil at the same time. This seems to work best.

Put the jar in a cool dark place for at least a week. At the end of this time, pour your new perfume creation into a perfume bottle, straining it first and enjoy the beautiful fragrances!

This recipe consists of essential oils, Vodka and spring or distilled water. For the best results, use a ratio of 20 to 30 percent essential oils, 70 to 80 percent Vodka and 5 percent water. Mix the essential oils of your choice with the Vodka, stirring well and put in a cool dark room for two days, making sure they're in a jar with a tightly fit lid.

After two days, add the water, stir again and let sit for another two days. Strain it through a coffee filter and store in a dark jar. Some popular essential oil choices are Jasmine, Lavender, Patchouli, Juniper or Ylang-Ylang.

Simplicity of Solid Perfumes

While filling up your little perfume containers with your favorite homemade perfume is easy, you'll find that making solid perfume is even easier.

Most of the supplies for making solid perfume can be found at a craft and health food stores. Here is a checklist to take to the store, so you can get busy making your favorite scent solid perfume.

- Small glass bowl for mixing
- Saucepan
- Stirring stick or straw
- Glass, stone or ceramic container for your perfume
- Essential oil of your choice
- Beeswax
- Almond or Jojoba oil or Vitamin E

Put one tablespoon of Almond or Jojoba oil and one tablespoon of wax in the small glass jar. Put about an inch of water in the saucepan and place the glass container with beeswax in it in the water. Bring the water in the saucepan to a boil to allow the wax to melt. When it's completed melted and liquid, remove it from the stove.

Add about eight to twelve drops of essential oils into the mixture. Stir it with a straw or stirring stick, allowing as little as possible to stick to the straw, so not to waste any of your precious perfume. Make sure it's thoroughly mixed.

Pour your liquefied wax into your glass or stone container and let it cool for at least 30 minutes. The mixture you've made will make about one half ounce of solid perfume. Once you get the hang of it, you'll want to make a larger amount.

When you're ready to use the perfume, all you have to do is rub your finger on the surface of the perfume and rub it on your neck, wrist or any place you desire. You'll find that solid perfume is fun to make and you'll want to experiment with many different fragrances. It's great for traveling and can be put in a small container of your choice and carried in your purse or glove compartment.

Different fragrances can be made for medicinal or special purposes. For instance, a mixture of Lavender or Chamomile essential oils makes a very relaxing scent. Applying solid perfume of Cypress or Cedarwood essential oil is great for a foot rub. You'll find that you not only will want to have several of these unique perfume scents in your home but they make great gifts as well.

Amaze Solid Perfume

Here's a nice solid perfume that you can carry with you in a pocket or purse to use when needed.

What You Will Need:
5 Drops St. John's Wort Essential Oil
10 Drops Cypress Essential Oil
10 Drops Rosemary Essential Oil
2 Teaspoons Beeswax Beads Oil
1 Tablespoon Sweet Almond Oil
1 Tablespoon Coconut Oil
Clean, empty Lipstick tubes or Small containers
Glass Measuring Cup

What To Do:

1. In a glass measuring cup, melt the Beeswax Beads and Coconut oil together in a microwave for 10 seconds or until melted.

2. Remove from the microwave and add Sweet Almond oil and essential oils in order according to each note.

3. Pour into ¼ ounce Lipstick/Balm tubes and close right away. Let cool completely.

4. To wear, apply solid perfume by rolling up a bit from the tube and rub on the inside of your wrists, behind your ears, elbows and knees.

5. This recipe will make five tubes. Recipe Variation: Add a few drops of Vitamin E oil as an antioxidant.

Summer Fling Solid Perfume

This solid perfume is great for summer as a refreshing fragrance. Carry in purse or pocket to dab on as needed.

What You Will Need:
1 Drop Ylang-Ylang Essential Oil
1 Drop Tangerine Essential Oil
2 Drops Jasmine Essential Oil
2 Drops Lavender Essential Oil
2 Drops Vanilla CO2 extract
3 Drops German Chamomile Essential Oil
2 Teaspoons Beeswax Beads
1 Tablespoon Coconut Oil
1 Tablespoon Sweet Almond Oil
5 Clean, Empty Lip Balm Tubes

What To Do:

1. Melt the Beeswax Beads and Coconut oil together. Remove from heat then add Sweet Almond oil and essential oils.

2. Pour into ¼ ounce lip balm tubes and close right away. Let cool completely.

3. To use your fragrance, roll the tube up a bit and rub on the inside of your wrist, behind your ears, elbows and/or knees.

4. This recipe makes approximately five tubes. Recipe Variation: You may also want to add a few drops of Vitamin E oil as an antioxidant.

More Perfume Recipes

Here are some simple instructions for creating your first batch of aromatherapy perfume:

What You Will Need:
1 Teaspoon Carrier Oil (Jojoba or Almond, etc.)
1 Teaspoon Alcohol (Vodka)
1 Glass Dropper Per Essential Oil
Essential Oils

What To Do:
1. Add the essential oils from your chosen recipe (below you will see a number of different recipes, with the quantities of essential oils you require for them).

2. Using a glass dropper, add one drop of essential oil at a time (pay attention to the notes of each essential oil and add in that order).

3. After adding each drop of essential oil to the rest of the mixture, the bottle should be shaken (remember to put the lid on first before shaking).

4. Once you have finished adding the last drops of essential oil and shaken, make sure the lid is on tightly, and store in a cool dark place for twelve days or more. However, each day you should remember to give the bottles a shake at least 3 times.

5. After twelve days you can begin to enjoy the aromatherapy perfume that you have made.

The first recipe below is specifically for those women who may suffer from nervous butterflies on their wedding day or another big event. This one will help the bride feel much more relaxed and calm on their big day.

Jitters
4 Drops Jasmine Essential Oil
2 Drops Lemon Essential Oil
1 Drop Patchouli Essential Oil

The following recipes have been designed to help produce a much more calming effect to the person using them. These perfumes will help you focus on your inner self, and provide you with a feeling of security, which will promote a feeling of total relaxation.

Tranquility
4 Drops Cedarwood Essential Oil
2 Drops Clary Sage Essential Oil
1 Drop Grapefruit Essential Oil
2 Drops Mandarin Essential Oil

Chill Out
2 Drops Grapefruit Essential Oil
2 Drops Patchouli Essential Oil
1 Drop Rose Essential Oil
3 Drops Vetiver Essential Oil
2 Drops Ylang-Ylang Essential Oil

Sleep Tight
2 Drops Bergamot Essential Oil
3 Drops Chamomile Essential Oil
2 Drops Marjoram Essential Oil
4 Drops Lavender Essential Oil

Serene
3 Drops Lavender Essential Oil
3 Drops Neroli Essential Oil
2 Drops Spearmint Essential Oil

The next recipes we are looking at will enhance a person's mood and feelings of wellbeing. These perfumes will help to relax and surround you with warmth, as well as a feeling of pure luxury for those special nights out or at home with your loved one.

Ardour
3 Drops Jasmine Essential Oil
3 Drops Neroli Essential Oil
4 Drops Orange Essential Oil

Devotion
1 Drop Clary Sage Essential Oil
3 Drops Patchouli Essential Oil
2 Drops Rose Essential Oil
4 Drops Rosewood Essential Oil

Tenderness
2 Drops Linden Blossom Essential Oil
3 Drops Lime Essential Oil
2 Drops Neroli Essential Oil
3 Drops Sandalwood Essential Oil

Zeal
4 Drops Melissa Essential Oil
2 Drops Rose Essential Oil
2 Drops Ylang-Ylang Essential Oil

Arabian Dusk
3 Drops Coriander Essential Oil
1 Drop Frankincense Essential Oil
3 Drops Juniper Essential Oil
4 Drops Orange Essential Oil

Motivation

1 Drop Frankincense Essential Oil
4 Drops Grapefruit Essential Oil
3 Drops Rosemary Essential Oil
2 Drops Spearmint Essential Oil

So now that you have a few recipes to consider, its time to get started making your own aromatherapy perfumes!

Moonlit Night Perfume

Imagine a moonlit trail of light reflected in quiet lake with only the sounds of crickets chirping and stars winking at you. Wear this perfume for a relaxing evening at home by the fireplace or peaceful stroll with a loved one.

What You Will Need:
2 Cups Distilled Water
4 Tablespoons Vodka or Perfumer's Alcohol
6 Drops Lavender Essential Oil
10 Drops Chamomile Essential Oil
Dark Glass Bottle

What To Do:

1. Add the Vodka first to the bottle. Add the essential oils in order according to each note.

2. Shake the mixture well then set aside for two to three weeks.

3. Add distilled water then set aside for one week. Shake once a day.

4. Store your perfume in a dark bottle or keep in a dark, cool place. Dab on pulse points for a long-lasting fragrance to enjoy throughout the day or evening.

Dignity Perfume
Feel good about yourself and live your dreams!

What You Will Need:
¼ Cup Vodka or Perfumer's Alcohol
2 Tablespoons Distilled Water
1 Tablespoon Glycerin
4 Drops Petitgrain Essential Oil
3 Drops Bergamot Essential Oil
2 Drops Basil Essential Oil
1 Drop Coriander Essential Oil
Glass Bottle

What To Do:

1. Add ¼ cup of alcohol to your bottle, followed by the essential oils. Let stand for 48 hours. Shake bottle each day for up to a month. The longer it sits, the stronger the fragrance will be.

2. After your perfume has sat for your preferred time, add distilled water. If your perfume is still too strong, add more water to get your desired strength.

3. To make your perfume last longer, add a tablespoon of glycerin to your blend. This colorless, neutral liquid will not affect the scent, but will help the other ingredients blend well.

Rosewater

Enjoy your garden year-round with the wonderful fragrance of Rosewater made with rose petals from your yard. Rosewater can be used in lotions, soaps, and potpourri – even candy!

What You Will Need:
½ Pound Fresh, Pesticide-Free Rose Petals
Boiling Water
Colander
Cheesecloth
String
Large Glass Bowl
Mason Jar With Lid

What To Do:

1. Pick your Rose petals fresh in the morning of your project.

2. Place Rose petals in a colander and rinse with cold water well.

3. Spread cheesecloth out then place Rose petals on top and tie to make a sack. Place sack in a large glass bowl then pour boiling water over sack of petals, just covering it.

4. Cover bowl with plastic wrap tightly, securing with a rubber band to hold in place.

5. Leave Roses in a bowl overnight to steep. In the morning, pour water into a glass mason jar. Be sure to squeeze cheesecloth to get all water out.

6. Replace jar with lid. Store your Rosewater in the refrigerator to keep fresh for up to two weeks. You can also store in freezer for six months.

Gulfport Breeze Perfume

Here is another simple recipe using soothing fragrances of Lavender, Chamomile and Valerian.

What You Will Need:
2 Cups Distilled Water
3 Tablespoons Vodka
5 Drops Lavender Essential Oil
10 Drops Chamomile Essential Oil
10 Drops Valerian Essential Oil

What To Do:

1. Mix all of these ingredients together in a bottle and shake it well.

2. Transfer the mixture to a dark colored bottle, and as with the previous recipe, allow the bottle to stand for 12 hours or more.

3. Once the bottle has stood for the recommended 12 hours, it can be used, and then stored in a cool dry place.

Rose Perfume

Using your fresh Rosewater just made, you can create your own romantic Rose perfume. The scent of this fragrance is timeless and will make a wonderful gift for a friend or family member.

What You Will Need:
2 Cups Rosewater
3 Tablespoons Vodka or Perfumer's Alcohol
10 Drops Rose Essential Oil
4 Drops Glycerin
Large Bowl
Glass Bottle

What To Do:

1. Measure out 2 cups of the cooled Rosewater into a large bowl.

2. Add Vodka, Rose essential oil and glycerin.

3. Stir the perfume and let it sit for a few minutes to develop its scent. Add a few drops of Rose essential oil if it is not as strong as you would like.

4. When you are satisfied with your perfume, pour into a perfume bottle and use daily.

Rose Garden Perfume

Imagine capturing the soft, delicate scent of your Rose garden in a perfume. In this formula, you will be making your own Rose essential oil from Roses in your garden then adding the rest of the ingredients to create your signature perfume.

What You Will Need:
4 Cups Rose Petals
1 Cup Sweet Almond Oil
1 Cup Distilled Water
5 Teaspoons Vodka or Perfumer's Alcohol
Small Bowl
Measuring Cup
Cheesecloth
Plastic Wrap
Funnel
Dark Glass Bottle

What To Do:

1. First, you will want to make your Rose essential oil. In a bowl, add your Rose petals and Sweet Almond oil and mash up using a wooden spoon or mortar.

2. Cover bowl with plastic wrap and allow the oil to sit overnight. In the morning, uncover and strain liquid using the cheesecloth and funnel into a glass container. Discard used Rose petals.

3. To make perfume, add alcohol, water and the Rose essential oil. Shake to mix well.

4. Allow your perfume to sit in a cool, dark place for 48 hours. Check for strength and leave for up to a month for a stronger fragrance.

Rose and Lavender Perfume

Here is an easy recipe for creating a light and airy fragrance.

What You Will Need:
1 Cup Vodka or Perfumer's Alcohol
6 Tablespoons Rosewater
1 Tablespoon Distilled Water
1 Drop Orange Essential Oil
1 Teaspoon Lavender Essential Oil
Glass Bottle
Saucepan
Wooden Spoon

What To Do:

1. Place Vodka and Rosewater in a saucepan to warm for one minute.

2. Add the essential oils in order according to each note then add the distilled water and stir using a wooden spoon.

3. Use a sterile funnel and pour liquid to a glass bottle. Let your perfume sit for 48-72 hours before using. Shake before applying to skin.

Lavender Perfume
This is a lovely fragrance that will sure to be a classic.

What You Will Need:
2 Cups Distilled Water
3 Tablespoons Vodka or Perfumer's Alcohol
10 Drops Lavender Essential Oil
8 Drops Chamomile Essential Oil
8 Drops Valerian Essential Oil
4 Drops Glycerin
Glass Bottle
Glass Measuring Cup

What To Do:

1. In a measuring cup, combine Vodka and distilled water.

2. Add essential oils to the measuring cup in order according to each note.

3. Place four drops of glycerin as a fixative to your perfume mixture to help retain its aroma.

4. Stir the mixture then test to see if you need to add any more of the essential oils, one drop at a time.

5. Pour your perfume into a glass bottle using a funnel. Replace lid on bottle and shake. Allow your perfume to sit in a dark cool place overnight before using.

Tender Mercies

This formula contains a collection of floral notes that will remind you of spring.

What You Will Need:
2 ½ Ounce Vodka or Perfumer's Alcohol
2 Tablespoons Distilled Water
4 Drops Carnation Essential Oil
3 Drops Juniper Essential Oil
3 Drops Ylang-Ylang Essential Oil
2 Drops Lavender Essential Oil
2 Drops Jasmine Essential Oil
Glass Bottle

What To Do:

1. Place your Vodka or Perfumer's Alcohol in your bottle. Add the essential oils in order according to each note. Shake to mix. Let blend sit for 48 hours.

2. Add distilled water and blend into mixture thoroughly. Let blend stand for another 48 hours up to a month of curing time. This time can vary depending on how strong you want your perfume to be.

3. If your formula is too strong, add more distilled water. Once your perfume has matured, pour through a coffee filter to strain off any sediment.

4. To apply your new perfume, dab on wrist pulse points and enjoy.

Sultans Pleasure

This one has a unique scent with a pleasant base note, but again, perfume scents are very subjective. Have fun experimenting with this one.

What You Will Need:
2 ½ Ounce Vodka or Perfumer's Alcohol
2 Tablespoons Distilled Water
2 Drops Patchouli Essential Oil
2 Drops Lavender Essential Oil
3 Drops Ylang-Ylang Essential Oil
1 Drop Jasmine Essential Oil
Glass Bottle

What To Do:

1. Place your Vodka or Perfumer's Alcohol in your bottle. Add the essential oils in order according to each note. Shake to mix. Let blend sit for 48 hours.

2. Add distilled water and blend into mixture thoroughly. Let blend stand for another 48 hours up to a month of curing time. This time can vary depending on how strong you want your perfume to be.

3. If your formula is too strong, add more distilled water. Once your perfume has matured, pour through a coffee filter to strain off any sediment. Pour into a glass bottle for storage.

4. To apply your new perfume, dab on wrist pulse points and enjoy.

Determination Perfume

Know what your want and make it happen.

What You Will Need:
¼ Cup Vodka or Perfumer's Alcohol
2 Tablespoons Distilled Water
1 Tablespoon Glycerin
3 Drops Frankincense Essential Oil
3 Drops Orange Essential Oil
2 Drops Onycha (Benzoin) Essential Oil
1 Drop Geranium Essential Oil
Glass Bottle

What To Do:

1. Add ¼ cup of alcohol to your bottle, followed by the essential oils in order according to each note. Let stand for 48 hours. Shake bottle each day for up to a month. The longer it sits, the stronger the fragrance will be.

2. After your perfume has sat for your preferred time, add distilled water. If your perfume is still too strong, add more water to get your desired strength.

3. To make your perfume last longer, add a tablespoon of glycerin to your blend. This colorless, neutral liquid will not affect the scent, but will help the other ingredients blend well.

Belief Perfume
Walk in faith and confidence of what your can achieve.

What You Will Need:
¼ Cup Vodka or Perfumer's Alcohol
2 Tablespoons Distilled Water
1 Tablespoon Glycerin
4 Drops Rosemary Essential Oil
3 Drops Myrtle Essential Oil
3 Drops Verbena Essential Oil
2 Drops Ginger Essential Oil
Glass Bottle

What To Do:

1. Add ¼ cup of alcohol to your bottle, followed by the essential oils in order according to each note. Let stand for 48 hours. Shake bottle each day for up to a month. The longer it sits, the stronger the fragrance will be.

2. After your perfume has sat for your preferred time, add distilled water. If your perfume is still too strong, add more water to get your desired strength.

3. To make your perfume last longer, add a table-spoon of glycerin to your blend. This colorless, neutral liquid will not affect the scent, but will help the other ingredients blend well.

Butterflies Perfume
Have courage and know you are doing what is right. .

What You Will Need:
¼ Cup Vodka or Perfumer's Alcohol
2 Tablespoons Distilled Water
1 Tablespoon Glycerin
4 Drops Jasmine Essential Oil
2 Drops Lemon Essential Oil
1 Drop Patchouli Essential Oil
Glass Bottle

What To Do:

1. Add ¼ cup of alcohol to your bottle, followed by the essential oils in order according to each note. Let stand for 48 hours. Shake bottle each day for up to a month. The longer it sits, the stronger the fragrance will be.

2. After your perfume has sat for your preferred time, add distilled water. If your perfume is still too strong, add more water to get your desired strength.

3. To make your perfume last longer, add a tablespoon of glycerin to your blend. This colorless, neutral liquid will not affect the scent, but will help the other ingredients blend well.

Fresh Squeezed Perfume

This one comes straight from the kitchen. All you need is vanilla extract and lemon.

What You Will Need:
1 Cup Distilled Water
¼ Cup Lemon Juice
6 Drops Vanilla Extract
Saucepan
Bottle

What To Do:

1. Mix the Vanilla extract and Lemon juice in a saucepan with one cup of water.

2. Bring liquid to a boil covered for a couple of minutes. Chill liquid in the refrigerator for 5 minutes then boil again.

3. Quickly remove from the burner, and pour liquid into a glass bottle and then into the refrigerator for 1 hour. After one hour, it is ready for use.

Passions Perfume

This recipe comes highly recommended as exotic and a sensual aroma for your senses. This recipe is sure to become one of your favorites.

What You Will Need:
½ Pint Vodka or Perfumer's Alcohol
3 Drops Passionflower Essential Oil
3 Drops Neroli Essential Oil
2 Drops Ylang-Ylang Essential Oil
Glass Bottle

What To Do:

1. Pour alcohol into glass bottle. Add essential oils in the correct order (base, middle, and top) shaking well after adding each oil.

2. Let stand in a dark, cool place for one week. Shake daily to blend.

3. When ready, dab on pulse points to wear your fragrance.

Rainforest Perfume

This fragrance will remind you of an oasis of pleasure.

What You Will Need:
2-3 Cups Distilled Water
3-4 Tablespoons Vodka or Perfumer's Alcohol
5-6 Drops Sandalwood Essential Oil
9-10 Drops Bergamot Essential Oil
Glass Bottle

What To Do:

1. Pour Vodka or perfumer's alcohol into a bottle. Shake well.

2. Add each essential oil in order of each note and shake well. Set aside for three weeks.

3. Add distilled water then set aside for another week. Shake once a day.

4. Store in dark bottles or keep in a cool dark place. Dab on pulse points to wear your new fragrance.

Start a Perfume Business

Now that you have begun to produce your own perfume and have given as gifts to your friends or family, you may want to begin to sell it to a wider audience.

One of the first things you will need to look at when making the decision on selling your own perfume is what to call it. You will then need to start looking for bottles in which you can put your finished perfume. Then you will need to design a label for inclusion on the bottle, and also consider the kind of packaging that you can present the perfume in.

When contemplating what sort of bottles to place your finished product in, you might want to think about vintage perfume bottles (but make sure they have been thoroughly sterilized). They will certainly provide you with an individual look that can not be found when buying perfumes that have been mass produced. Just take a wander around your local antique shops or bric-a-brac shop, and you will soon find a wealth of different perfume bottles that you could use.

The best place to start when you are considering selling your own perfume is to do a search on the internet. There are many sites and companies which will provide you with all the necessary information you need in order to start up.

However, you should be prepared to make some financial outlays in order to get the business started. For instance, you will need to factor in such costs as the purchase of all the ingredients for making the perfume, and the bottles that you will be putting the finished product into.

Other costs that you will need to include are the production of the labels that will be affixed to your finished product's bottles, and the cost of the packaging/box that you will use.

When first selling your product, it is advisable that you keep a record of all of your outgoing expenses so that you can price your perfume accordingly. The usual pricing equation is four times the price of the materials it costs you to manufacture your product. So say it has cost you $5 to produce each bottle, you should probably sell it for at least $20. Don't forget to figure in the cost of your time as well.

One of the best ways of selling your own perfume is through word of mouth of friends and family. However, for a small outlay, you could actually set up your own website and sell it online.

If you are not sure how to go about setting up a website, you will find many people who are able to help online. There are free services as well as forums where professionals will assist you at no charge. They will also help with the marketing and promotion of the product you have to offer. Begin by doing a search on the internet and looking for "starting a small web business". You will soon find a whole list of sites that are willing to assist you.

So, as you can see, making perfume is not only easy and provides you with a new skill, but it can also be profitable too.

Some of the most expensive perfumes available on the market cost next to nothing to produce and now you can make your own perfume for just a few dollars. Research has shown that you can actually make a 100 bottles of perfume for less than $300, and then, resell them for up to $50 each.

At one time when people were considering making their own perfume it was very difficult to find all of the ingredients, as well as packaging (bottles, spray nozzles etc). Now with the internet, this has all changed. Today you can browse the web to find the necessary ingredients at reasonable prices and have them delivered directly to your door. You can also find some ingredients at a local health food store or craft store.

Here is a simple checklist of "To Do's" to consider before you commence a perfume business:

1.   First, you will want to come up with a name for your fragrance and perfume brand. Try to come up with something catchy that people will remember. Once you have a name, you will need to design a label (simple artwork works best).

2.   Second, make a list of all of the supplies and ingredients you will need.

3.   Third, search online for the best types of glass bottles (lids and pumps too) for putting your perfume in. Spend time on this step, so you can make your product look professional.

4.   Fourth, find recipes online that you can practice making and purchase the ingredients you will need to create your perfume. Take a few days making your choices. It is important you do as much research as possible on which ones will work best for you.

5.   Once you have received your ingredients, you will want to work in a sterile environment when blending your oils and pouring into the perfume bottles you have chosen.

6. Finally, look for a creative way to present the finished product to customers… it may be in a box, or you may find a much more unique way to do this.

As you can see, starting your own perfume company is a simple process. Even if you are only making perfume for your own personal use or as a gift for a loved one or friend, it is something you will enjoy doing. Not only that, but creating your own perfume boosts confidence as you learn a new skill.

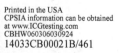
Printed in the USA
CPSIA information can be obtained
at www.ICGtesting.com
CBHW060306030924
14033CB00021B/461